A YEAR OF INTENTIONAL LIVING

Prepare Your Mind for a Phenomenal Year

By: Dr. Josiane Joseph

A Year of Intentional Living

Text, illustrations, and book's cover are Copyright © 2025 by Josiane Joseph of Double Doc J LLC. All Rights Reserved.

No portion of this book may be reproduced, stored, or transmitted in any form or by any means, including photocopy, recording, or any information retrieval system, without written permission from author and publisher.

Cover Art
Designed by Patricia Belfort. Used with permission and gratitude.

Bulk Purchases
Books are available at special discounts when purchased in bulk. Visit doubledocj.com for inquiries.

Disclaimer
The author has made every effort to ensure the accuracy of contact information at the time of publication. However, neither the author nor publisher assumes responsibility for any errors or changes after publication.

For permission requests, please contact:

Double Doc J LLC
DoubleDocJ.com

All trademarks, product names, and company names are the property of their respective owners.

This book is dedicated to those who strive to live and be better. A healthier world begins with you.

Contents

PART I
Introduction   1

PART II
1. Celebrate Remarkable Gifts   4
2. Food for Health   12
3. Major Accomplishments   20
4. Focus on Forgiveness   28
5. Read Daily   36
6. Send Thanks   44
7. Sing Daily   48
8. Rise Early   56
9. Picture This   64
10: Walk Daily   72
11. Daily Affirmations   80
12. Clean Up   88
13. Share Laughter   96
14. Morning Meditation   104
15. Draw Your Dreams   112
16. Heart for Health   120
17. Disown Fears   128
18. Celebrate Mini Gifts   136
19. No Complaints   144
20. Breath Daily   152
21. Outside is Ours   160
22. Compliment Daily   168
23. Healthy Hobbies   176
24. Our Children   184
25. Focus on Objects   192
26. Rest Daily   200
27. Eat Vegetables   208
28. Dance Daily   216

29. Share Love	224
30. Good News Only	232
31. Notice Your Body	240
32. Gift Giving	248
33. Wealth in Water	256
34. Sleep Well	264
35. Celebrate Life	272
36. Be With Friends	280
37. Values	288
38. In the Clouds	296
39. Great Gifts	304
40. Exercise	312
41. Self-Forgiveness	320
42. Smiles	328
43. Sense of Thanks	336
44. Eat for Enrichment	344
45. Greet Yourself	352
46. Reframe the Negative	360
47. Play Daily	368
48. Purposeful Reading	376
49. Ask It	384
50. Positive Routine	392
51. Sleep Grateful	400
52. Celebrate Success	408
PART III Conclusion	417
a. Color Daily	419
b. Laugh Daily	420
c. Turtle Detection	421
d. Dream Daily	422
Acknowledgements	423

Part I

Introduction

Have you ever been jolted by an unexpected event like being hit by a bus, a semi-truck, or an older lady on a scooter? Afterward, you might recognize that every day is a gift. Whether you are familiar with trauma or seeking focus, contentment, or peace, you have made a meaningful decision in choosing this book.

As we accept more responsibilities, we may forget to reflect on the wealth of experiences we get to have. There is divinity in each moment and connection with other living beings or objects. Life is better when we acknowledge what is sacred and nourish our minds—an essential component of our existence.

For that goal, this book was created. In it, you will discover an accessible guide to pause, reflect, and reconnect with what matters. Themes of gratitude, generosity, vision, affirmations, routines, and holistic health will ground you on this 52-week journey. Thank you for taking this step to prioritize your well-being.

Each week, I introduce a practice for you to explore. Some of these may be familiar to you and important health principles are represented. (It is okay to skip one and use alternatives available in Part III of the book.) To reap the most benefit, avoid missing more than two consecutive days of any practice. Consistency will take you far.

Give yourself the best opportunity for growth by committing to your improvement. Keep in mind that life is about progress, not perfection. Approach each task with a focus on personal wellness. Modify and interpret the prompts to support your goals.

For most of these exercises, finding a quiet space to ponder may be beneficial. Alternatively, you could play calming music to drown out distractions. Remember, preparation and positive expectations are foundational principles of success.

Wellness is not just an individual journey—it is a mission we share with others. Without an inquisitive mindset, it is challenging to understand where and what we need to grow. This book offers a range of exercises for experimenting or choosing for regular use.

Many of these exercises are more impactful if you ask for advice. If others are seeking peace or contentment they may join you on your journey.

Writing is an effective tool to organize your thoughts while exploring the natural world. It also gives you a record for future reference. Dedicate at least 15 minutes per day for each task and writing. Even if it is just one sentence or a few words, write daily. A small commitment can change your life.

As you go through each exercise, take time to reflect. Consider these questions: Who does this activity remind me of? What are the challenges? When was the last time I experienced something like this? Where is my mind with this practice? Why might this be beneficial for me? How do I feel? There are questions associated with prompts but refer back to these as needed to write daily.

While the instructions suggest committing to a practice for 7 days, it typically takes a couple of weeks to form a habit. If you want to integrate a practice into your routine, consider doing a task for 3-6 weeks.

Even if our circumstances appear bleak, we can affirm our hope for our futures today. This will be a phenomenal year, and we will be well.

Part II

1. Celebrate Remarkable Gifts

Millions of sperm race to an egg during conception. Only one can be successful in fertilization. Incredibly, we beat the odds before and at birth. To be born is a gift. With birth, many of us are given family, shelter, regular food, health, a mind, and breath. These are examples of extraordinary gifts or items that support our existence.

As you move through the day, reflect on remarkable gifts. Use the following space to write down five remarkable gifts today and continue doing so for the next six days.

After creating your list, describe what it means to be alive. What does a full life look like to you? Who helps you to have what you need to thrive? Have there been times when you did not have these gifts? Reflect on those moments and the impact they had on you. Consider the experiences of others who may lack these essential gifts and how their life differs. What emotions do these reflections evoke for you?

Date: _____ Day 1 of 7

1.
2.
3.
4.
5.

Date: _____ Day 2 of 7

1.
2.
3.
4.
5.

Date: _____ Day 3 of 7

1.
2.
3.
4.
5.

Date: _____ Day 4 of 7

1.
2.
3.
4.
5.

Date: _____ Day 5 of 7

1.
2.
3.
4.
5.

Date: _____ Day 6 of 7

1.
2.
3.
4.
5.

Date: _____ Day 7 of 7 ☺

1.
2.
3.
4.
5.

2. Food for Health

Do squirrels in Florida hibernate? No. Yet you will still find them storing and hiding food. Why? Because these habits serve them in a different season and environment.

Similarly, habits we form can be beneficial, neutral, or harmful. They warrant regular questioning and adjusting where possible.

Our food habits affect our health thereby impacting our minds and remaining days. Our resources limit our diet options.

If we get to choose, why not adjust for better health? Resources for healthier eating might suggest a reduction of processed foods (such as individually packaged snacks or candies), solid oils, cured meats, red meat, items with high sugar content (such as sodas, ice creams, juices, and certain cereals), alcohol, energy drinks, and bread.

For one week, avoid one unhealthy food or food group. Choose one of the examples above or focus on a habit you would like to break. Remember, one good choice is better than no good choice.

Dedicate this sacrifice to honoring your mind and body. As you make this commitment, journal about your vision for a healthier you. Reflect on the challenges and your plans to overcome them.

Date: _____ Day 1 of 7

I am avoiding:

Date: _____ Day 2 of 7

Date: _____ Day 3 of 7

Date: _____ Day 4 of 7

Date: _____ Day 5 of 7

Date: _____ Day 6 of 7

Date: _____ Day 7 of 7 ☺

3. Major Accomplishments

By a decade of life, many of us have stored precious memories of overcoming challenges that appeared insurmountable.

Examples of accomplishments may be earning a degree, advancing in a career, purchasing a house, achieving a health goal, or making a new meaningful connection. Sometimes, a major success may be getting up and facing the day.

We have succeeded on numerous occasions when failure was possible. Every victory is a testament to our perseverance and growth. Cherish the memories of these triumphs.

For the next seven days (starting today), identify one major accomplishment daily. Reflect on what it took to achieve your goal. What did you learn? Embrace how it changed your life. Consider how it impacted the lives of others. Write down your thoughts regarding each major accomplishment daily.

After reviewing your great works, reaffirm your strength by saying and writing: "I HAVE what it takes for success!"

Date: _____ Day 1 of 7

Accomplishment:

_____
_____
_____
_____
_____
_____
_____
_____
_____
_____
_____
_____
_____
_____
_____
_____
_____
_____
_____

Affirmation:

_____
_____

Date: _____ Day 2 of 7

Accomplishment:
_____
_____
_____
_____
_____
_____
_____
_____
_____
_____
_____
_____
_____
_____
_____
_____
_____
_____
_____
_____
_____
_____

Affirmation:
_____
_____

Date: _____ Day 3 of 7

Accomplishment:
_____
_____
_____
_____
_____
_____
_____
_____
_____
_____
_____
_____
_____
_____
_____
_____
_____
_____
_____

Affirmation:
_____
_____

Date: _____ Day 4 of 7

Accomplishment:
_____
_____
_____
_____
_____
_____
_____
_____
_____
_____
_____
_____
_____
_____
_____
_____
_____
_____
_____
_____

Affirmation:
_____
_____

Date: _____ Day 5 of 7

Accomplishment:
_____
_____
_____
_____
_____
_____
_____
_____
_____
_____
_____
_____
_____
_____
_____
_____
_____
_____
_____
_____
_____

Affirmation:
_____
_____

Date: _____ Day 6 of 7

Accomplishment:

Affirmation:

Date: _____ Day 7 of 7 ☺

Accomplishment:
_____
_____
_____
_____
_____
_____
_____
_____
_____
_____
_____
_____
_____
_____
_____
_____
_____
_____
_____
_____

Affirmation:
_____
_____

4. Focus on Forgiveness

There are over eight billion people on one Earth, and, unfortunately, not all of them will treat us kindly. A trap whose only use is to clutter the mind is perseverating on past injustices. Negative thoughts about betrayals may keep us stuck and drain our energy. They rarely serve our values. Even if you never receive an apology, choosing forgiveness is freeing.

Forgiveness is prioritizing yourself by releasing the emotional burden associated with past events. Forgiveness is a choice and does not require the restoration of a relationship. It does not mend trust or excuse misdeeds. But over time, forgiveness creates space in your mind for great thoughts that will nourish you.

Each day, reflect on one instance of betrayal. Write a letter to that person—there is no need to send it. Write what occurred. Describe how it made you feel. Then write that you release the power those actions have over you. Let your letter declare your intention to move on for peace and greatness.

Forgiveness can be a process that takes time. That is okay. Either forgive one instance a day or take the time needed to forgive. Journal daily and affirm personal strength and self-love that allows for forgiveness (with boundaries).

Try to reframe the experience. Instead of allowing negative memories, choose to let go. Focus on purpose and progress. Remind yourself of lessons learned or the good obtained from that connection. Write about hopes for the future. Distance yourself from the hurt. Live in freedom.

Date: _____ Day 1 of 7

Date: _____ Day 2 of 7

Date: _____ Day 3 of 7

Date: _____ Day 4 of 7

Date: _____ Day 5 of 7

Date: _____ Day 6 of 7

Date: _____ Day 7 of 7 ☺

5. Read Daily

Reading exercises our minds. There is a wealth of information available to those who seek it. We can find newspapers, books, magazines, journal articles, and applications containing knowledge. Role models, librarians, search engines, and social media may give us suggestions.

This week, choose some form of literature. Get a library card if you do not have one. (That may take a day.) Then, read for at least 30 minutes per day for at least six days. Try for a consistent time daily.

As you read, notice the print on the page or device. Does the media have a smell? Are there memories connected to your choice? Have you read anything similar? Does this information remind you of someone? What, in your life, is related to the information? How do you feel while reading the words? Are there words that draw you in the text? Can you visualize what is described? Who is the author? How can you relate to the writer?

Reflect on these questions and journal about your thoughts.

Date: _____ Day 1 of 7

Reading choice:

Date: _____ Day 2 of 7

Date: _____ Day 3 of 7

Date: _____ Day 4 of 7

Date: _____ Day 5 of 7

Date: _____ Day 6 of 7

Date: _____ Day 7 of 7 ☺

6. Send Thanks

After receiving a present, we may say "thank you." But "thank yous" can also be gifts. Who doesn't appreciate gratitude from those around them? Genuine gratitude strengthens shared bonds.

Your circle may build or break you. Positive influence is worth celebrating. Whether someone makes you laugh or your load lighter, they deserve acknowledgment.

This week, purpose yourself to give tangible thanks. Choose "Thank You" cards. (There are affordable options online or in dollar stores.) Write 1-2 notes to people expressing your appreciation for their help or encouragement. Thank them for their patience if you were late or for other actions that improved your life.

The people around you are your people. Take ownership of the fact that unknown circumstances placed them before you. Help them understand that their existence is impactful while you have them. Remember, you reap what you sow. Plan for your harvest of gratitude.

Reflect on your feelings after giving your note. How did the recipient respond to you? Why did you choose the cards you are sending?

Date: _____ Day 1 of 7

Reason for card choice: _____
_____
_____
_____
_____

Date: _____ Day 2 of 7

Who did you thank: _____
_____
_____
_____
_____

Date: _____ Day 3 of 7

Who did you thank: _____
_____
_____
_____
_____

Date: _____ Day 4 of 7

Who did you thank:
_____
_____
_____
_____

Date: _____ Day 5 of 7

Who did you thank:
_____
_____
_____
_____

Date: _____ Day 6 of 7

Who did you thank:
_____
_____
_____
_____

Date: _____ Day 7 of 7 ☺

Reflect on responses and associated feelings
Who did you thank:

7. Sing Daily

Music is in unexpected places. The ability to hear is a great gift, not given to everyone, and can diminish over the course of life. Our voices are instruments; even if we prefer listening to others more than our own, we can still celebrate the music we enjoy. By using our instrument every day, we can uplift ourselves.

For the next seven days, sing at least once per day. Choose upbeat positive messages or hum to instrumentals.

Make a joyful noise while driving, in the shower, or cooking. Let the sound of your unique gift ring out. Change the way the song sounds. Sing it slowly or with different emotions.

Did someone join you in the song? Why did you choose that melody? How does music make you feel? Does it inspire you to dance? What kind of music do you prefer? Why? Write.

Date: _____ Day 1 of 7

Date: _____ Day 2 of 7

Date: _____ Day 3 of 7

Date: _____ Day 4 of 7

Date: _____ Day 5 of 7

Date: _____ Day 6 of 7

Date: _____ Day 7 of 7 ☺

8. Rise Early

No one knows for certain how much time we are gifted. If you ever felt there was insufficient time in the day, waking up earlier may be your ticket to purpose.

To get the most out of each day, we should start by attending to our minds. That looks different for everyone.

Exercise, meditation, activities for joy, discussions with loved ones, prayer, musical engagement, and/or affirmations are investments made possible if we get up just 30 minutes earlier than usual.

For the next six days, wake up earlier to give your mind the care it needs. Decide how that time will look today, and write down your plan. Write about challenges with this task as you plan and rise earlier.

Remember to avoid missing more than two consecutive days of this practice as you decide what would allow you to start the day off in a meaningful way.

Date: _____ Day 1 of 7

Morning plan:

Date: _____ Day 2 of 7

Date: _____ Day 3 of 7

Date: _____ Day 4 of 7

Date: _____ Day 5 of 7

Date: _____ Day 6 of 7

Date: _____ Day 7 of 7 ☺

9. Picture This

Bald eagles have exceptional eyesight, with visual acuity several times better than humans. They see in ways we will never see, and it helps them to live as birds of prey. But we have an advantage to keep seeing what we've seen.

Nowadays technology allows us to document every aspect of life: food, scenery, rooms, hobbies, etc. Incredibly, we can instantly capture memories and store them long-term. Our days are filled with tasks, many of which we have done before. While they may seem routine, our ability to continue doing them is a gift.

Think (and write) of what you formerly could do but no longer have that capacity. The mundane is precious. For the next seven days, take a picture of regular activities. Invite others to join you in photos. Create memories.

Did you share that moment with someone? Can you recall learning to perform the task in the picture? Write about why you chose that picture and what you might think when you see that image later.

Who knows what life will bring? Images help to remind us of times we will never see again. Cherish the mundane.

Date: _____ Day 1 of 7

Describe and reflect on picture

Date: _____ Day 2 of 7

Describe and reflect on picture

Date: _____ Day 3 of 7

Describe and reflect on picture

Date: _____ Day 4 of 7

Describe and reflect on picture

Date: _____ Day 5 of 7

Describe and reflect on picture

Date: _____ Day 6 of 7

Describe and reflect on picture

Date: _____ Day 7 of 7 ☺

Describe and reflect on picture

10: Walk Daily

Our minds are a product of our brains. Our brains, inside our bodies, are developed by our environment and practices. When we consider if we will exercise, we should consider that we do it to nourish our minds.

Exercise enhances flow to the brain and adjusts hormonal release. Valuing our minds means valuing regular exercise. A desire for mental clarity or emotional regulation should prompt the development of an exercise plan.

As possible, walk for a minimum of 30 minutes per day. Walk daily for at least seven days. During your walk, rest your mind. Tell thoughts against peace to leave and focus on positive alternatives. If music helps, choose wisely. Consider only encouraging, calming, and positive music.

If walking is already a habit, ramp up the pace or invite friends. Try different venues such as the park, beach, gym, or mall.

Be observant and careful. What wildlife is sharing these spaces with you? Are there people? Write about what you notice after your walk.

Date: _____ Day 1 of 7

Date: _____ Day 2 of 7

Date: _____ Day 3 of 7

Date: _____ Day 4 of 7

Date: _____ Day 5 of 7

Date: _____ Day 6 of 7

Date: _____ Day 7 of 7 ☺

11. Daily Affirmations

Have you ever seen a pair of Northern Cardinals whirling through the sky in their scarlet dressings? Though beautiful, they are aggressive as their fiery color suggests. They are known to fight their own image. Yet, as an example of loyalty, they mate for life.

While existing, we have the privilege of being companions to ourselves. Sometimes we battle with a habit of focusing on areas for improvement. Though it is honorable to be honest with yourself, an attitude of negativity, shame, or defeat detracts from purpose.

A person who thinks and speaks well of you is wonderful to be around. As your most consistent companion, you can encourage and be gentle with yourself.

Determine three kind phrases that you need to hear. Write them down and say them to yourself daily. Speak them boldly. Repeat them multiple times a day. Hear them and accept them as a loving gift.

As you write, reflect on personal traits that you admire. Do the people around you model them? How can you get to a place of admiring yourself and the people surrounding you?

Date: _____ Day 1 of 7

1.

2.

3.

Date: _____ Day 2 of 7

1.

2.

3.

Date: _____ Day 3 of 7

1.

2.

3.

Date: _____ Day 4 of 7

1. _____

2. _____

3. _____

Date: _____ Day 5 of 7

1.

2.

3.

Date: _____ Day 6 of 7

1.

2.

3.

Date: _____ Day 7 of 7 ☺

1. _____

2. _____

3. _____

12. Clean Up

Just as the people around us influence our being, the environment we live in defines us.

What does your environment say about you? Is it chaotic? Is it colorless? Does the atmosphere provoke peace, fun, love, welcome, or joy? You deserve a nurturing environment.

A disorganized, filthy, and impersonal home may reflect internal status. To cultivate peace within, create it in your environment.

For the next seven days, examine your space and organize it. Take at least one step towards a clear/comfortable home. Empty the sink and counters of dishes or designate 15 minutes per day to pick up around the house. (Do you need to get rid of items?)

If clutter is not the problem, then consider refreshing your space with new décor or rearrangements. (Do not live out of boxes or luggage.) Make your space homey.

Act on your thoughts as they arise because they will bring you good. Resist the temptation to do it later, tell yourself "Do it now." Reduce the stimulation of your mind by reducing the clutter in your environment.

Write about your state of mind and how your different environments have contributed to it. You CAN improve your environment and your mind.

Date: _____ Day 1 of 7

Date: _____ Day 2 of 7

Date: _____ Day 3 of 7

Date: _____ Day 4 of 7

Date: _____ Day 5 of 7

Date: _____ Day 6 of 7

Date: _____ Day 7 of 7 ☺

13. Share Laughter

Children are talented laughers. Their squeaky cackles can fill the room and bring smiles to everyone around. They laugh at the silliest ideas and seem to do it wholeheartedly. Laughs are contagious.

When was the last time you had a good laugh? Or made someone around you laugh? There are oodles of jokes and anecdotes to share to get the job done.

This week, let's give the children a run for their money and plan to laugh with someone at least once per day. Tell jokes, make faces, or spontaneously dance. Enjoy each day. Laugh.

Write about each new experience laughing. Reflect on past experiences where laughter was part of the atmosphere. Who do you laugh with the most?

Date: _____ Day 1 of 7

Date: _____ Day 2 of 7

Date: _____ Day 3 of 7

Date: _____ Day 4 of 7

Date: _____ Day 5 of 7

Date: _____ Day 6 of 7

Date: _____ Day 7 of 7 ☺

14. Morning Meditation

Our bodies need rest. In sync with our bodies is our mind which coordinates everything while alert and unconscious. For its efforts, our minds deserve a dedicated time of peace. Meditation allows that.

All it takes is to empty the mind of random thoughts and focus. Find a quiet and comfortable space. Focus on deep belly breathing. Exhale should be roughly twice as lengthy as inhale. Count the seconds for each breathing phase.

Allow thoughts to come with no judgment or emotional reaction. Set a goal of 20 minutes of meditation. As necessary, start with shorter periods of up to 10 minutes with short breaks and progressively lengthen your sessions. (Applications may be helpful for meditation.)

Plan for the meditation by choosing a time you will adhere to. It may help to associate it with a routine activity, such as combing your hair.

Journal after each meditation. Consider what helped you to stay focused and what was distracting.

Date: _____ Day 1 of 7

Date: _____ Day 2 of 7

Date: _____ Day 3 of 7

Date: _____ Day 4 of 7

Date: _____ Day 5 of 7

Date: _____ Day 6 of 7

Date: _____ Day 7 of 7 ☺

15. Draw Your Dreams

It is said that our brains cannot decipher between reality and what is seen. Images repeatedly focused on become true.

You know the desires of your heart, so why not make them real in a simple way? Reflect on what you hope to live for and with in the future.

Draw (in the following space) or use technology to create images that depict your desires. Focus on one theme or goal each day (for example, relationships, health, career, purchases, or personal development). Fill in the details. Place them where you can see them daily.

For seven days write as if your desires are reality. Write about gratitude for their existence. Consider who and what life events have shaped your dreams. Do you know people who encourage you to keep your hopes alive? What steps can you take to build your community and progress toward your dreams? A good decision can change your life; the images you focus on can help you to make one.

Date: _____ Day 1 of 7

Date: _____ Day 2 of 7

Date: _____ Day 3 of 7

Date: _____ Day 4 of 7

Date: _____ Day 5 of 7

Date: _____ Day 6 of 7

Date: _____ Day 7 of 7 ☺

16. Heart for Health

Out of our hearts stream rivers of life. For most of us, it is constantly working, feeding our minds and every other critical portion of our bodies that supports our existence. It sits at our core and creates music to reassure us of its active presence. Our hearts work for us, and we should make the job easier for them. Exercise that accelerates our heartbeat is beneficial to most people.

As you are able, run, dance, jump rope, swim, or do other activities to give your heart the practice and attention it deserves. Do at least 30 minutes of cardio exercise daily for the next seven days.

Journal about how your body and mind respond. Can you feel the pulses of blood? Are you out of breath? What is the difficulty level of your workout? What are your goals for your heart health? How do you feel about your weekly activity levels? What motivates you to exercise? Write.

Date: _____ Day 1 of 7

Date: _____ Day 2 of 7

Date: _____ Day 3 of 7

Date: _____ Day 4 of 7

Date: _____ Day 5 of 7

Date: _____ Day 6 of 7

Date: _____ Day 7 of 7 ☺

17. Disown Fears

Emotions are controllable. As we mature, we may develop ways of coping with negative feelings and inadvertently relinquish control. Fear can lead to maladaptive behavior. It keeps us from purposeful actions and events, sometimes without us recognizing the loss. The good news is that we can overcome our barriers—fear is no exception.

Whether it is fear of failure, letting go, rejection, financial loss, change, or the unknown, we can acknowledge it and remove its power. Taking back our power allows us to achieve what we value.

Confronting fear allows us to focus on priorities. When making decisions we must consider if we are honoring our fears or living a full life. Even a small step towards moving beyond fear is greater than no action at all.

Next time you notice yourself freezing up, procrastinating, avoiding something positive, dwelling on uncontrollable circumstances, or reacting out of your norm it may be because of fear. Consider how it might hinder you and take strides to move past it. Words have power so you can work through these feelings aloud by starting with a simple phrase like:

"Fear has no hold on me."

This week, consider goals that fear interferes with. Write about what you would gain from achieving the goals. What steps can you take towards your goal? What obstacles will you face? Are they real? What strategies can you employ to overcome them? Who might be a resource to move past the blockage? Redirect any negative thoughts (exchange them for thoughts of what you love and goals for the future). Write about the process.

Date: _____ Day 1 of 7

Date: _____ Day 2 of 7

Date: _____ Day 3 of 7

Date: _____ Day 4 of 7

Date: _____ Day 5 of 7

Date: _____ Day 6 of 7

Date: _____ Day 7 of 7 ☺

18. Celebrate Mini Gifts

If you see a female peacock, it may be difficult to recognize. The pictures typically shown are of the males with their lengthy iridescent plumes whose primary role is decoration to attract a partner. Peacocks do not need flashy feathers but it's nice that some can display them.

Similarly, there are many items we can live without, but they improve our experiences. Some examples include a smile, a joke, delicious food, or a standard household device that makes life easier. It could also be the internet, mail services, phones, or games.

Make a list of seven mini gifts daily. Write about how they enhance your life. How did you obtain those items? Are they replaceable? What do they add to your days? Reflecting on mini gifts in life fosters a beneficial habit of celebration.

Date: _____ Day 1 of 7

1.
2.
3.
4.
5.
6.
7.

Date: _____ Day 2 of 7

1.
2.
3.
4.
5.
6.
7.

Date: _____ Day 3 of 7

1.
2.
3.
4.
5.
6.
7.

Date: _____ Day 4 of 7

1.
2.
3.
4.
5.
6.
7.

Date: _____ Day 5 of 7

1.
2.
3.
4.
5.
6.
7.

Date: _____ Day 6 of 7

1.
2.
3.
4.
5.
6.
7.

Date: _____ Day 7 of 7 ☺

1.
2.
3.
4.
5.
6.
7.

19. No Complaints

Each day is a gift full of surprises and challenges. How we respond to them is our choice. While we may be influenced by our environment, it is up to us whether we relish our days. One obstacle preventing the proper acceptance of the gift of time is complaints.

It is easy to gripe about any inconvenience. But what do we gain from complaining (outside of annoyance)? What if, instead, we chose kind, supportive, and encouraging phrases to bring our minds joy and rest?

Take rain, for example. For folks living in cities, it may be inconvenient, but to a farmer, it is a sign of an upcoming harvest. We could all adopt that sign for ourselves. Claim a harvest every time it rains. We eat the fruit of the Earth, and we have other areas where this symbol of impending prosperity could encourage us.

During the next seven days, catch every complaint and transform it into a compliment or encouragement. Or deny complaints your voice.

Instead of complaining about traffic, celebrate the ability to travel on paved roads. Instead of complaining about a job, celebrate the income and remind yourself that it is a stepping stone to the next stage of life. (Make plans for that life and recognize that your experiences now will be a foundation for your dreams.)

Open yourself up to more gifts by recognizing and honoring gifts you have such as time, means of survival, and people. Write.

Date: _____ Day 1 of 7

Date: _____ Day 2 of 7

Date: _____ Day 3 of 7

Date: _____ Day 4 of 7

Date: _____ Day 5 of 7

Date: _____ Day 6 of 7

Date: _____ Day 7 of 7 ☺

20. Breath Daily

Breathing changes under duress. It may be short and shallow, or it may increase in frequency. We may not even notice these changes until we take a moment to examine our breaths. Are we taking restful breaths or shortchanging ourselves (and our minds) of oxygen exchange?

For the next seven days, spend at least 10 minutes focusing on breathing. Practice breathing with your diaphragm. (Belly moves rather than chest/shoulders.) As you are able, take slow deep breaths, and count during the inhale. Exhale slowly and for a longer period than inhale, count then too. Inhale through the nose and exhale through the mouth.

How does it feel to breathe this way? How is your mood? Is this task challenging? Why? How can you improve throughout the week? Are there thoughts intruding? In what ways can focusing on your breathing help you? Write.

Date: _____ Day 1 of 7

Date: _____ Day 2 of 7

Date: _____ Day 3 of 7

Date: _____ Day 4 of 7

Date: _____ Day 5 of 7

Date: _____ Day 6 of 7

Date: _____ Day 7 of 7 ☺

21. Outside is Ours

We are of the Earth, as is everything we engage with. It is remarkable that air we breathe out, plants breathe in, and they use it to color the world. Who can fathom even a fraction of the incredible offerings of the Earth?

For this week, take proper safety precautions, and plan an outside activity. Write about the preparations and feelings associated with the plans. Reflect on the gifts of the Earth.

Who will be with you for this endeavor? Will this be an activity you experienced before or are you trying something new? Purpose yourself to be amazed about what you see around you daily and while engaging in the activity. Write about what amazes you on the Earth (even if it is not something you saw recently).

Date: _____ Day 1 of 7

Date: _____ Day 2 of 7

Date: _____ Day 3 of 7

Date: _____ Day 4 of 7

Date: _____ Day 5 of 7

Date: _____ Day 6 of 7

Date: _____ Day 7 of 7 ☺

22. Compliment Daily

Villages, cities, countries, continents, and oceans separate so many of us. Yet unfathomable circumstances have placed some right beside us. That connection is divine.

Celebrate that understanding and help a peer celebrate the connection too by giving well-meaning compliments. These should not highlight what people cannot easily change (such as body form). Suggestions are: mind, garments, work, personality, use of language, or character traits.

Sometimes we are unaware of the impact our words have on others. Help others to see what you notice and appreciate by sharing a daily compliment for the next seven days.

Write about the experience of sharing compliments and about the compliments you have received. Consider ways that your words have impacted your relationships.

Date: _____ Day 1 of 7

Date: _____ Day 2 of 7

Date: _____ Day 3 of 7

Date: _____ Day 4 of 7

Date: _____ Day 5 of 7

Date: _____ Day 6 of 7

Date: _____ Day 7 of 7 ☺

23. Healthy Hobbies

Consider that the world was only covered in nature and creatures. Then people paved and shaped the landscape into towns, cities, and countries. We made something out of everything. Creativity is who we are.

Creativity, aside from being a feature of our identity, stimulates the mind. We love the beautiful, fun, mind-boggling, and delicious experiences of this world. As we fulfill responsibilities, sometimes creativity is pushed off to the wayside. For the sake of our minds, it is time to pull it back to the forefront.

This week be creative. Think about what brings you joy. What makes you smile? What do you like to talk about? Is it puzzles, sudoku, math, languages, sewing, knitting, cooking, baking, painting, or crosswords?

Pick a task and do it for at least 15-30 minutes daily. Write about the experience. Are you learning something new? Are there muscles at work that you don't regularly use? Write.

Date: _____ Day 1 of 7

Date: _____ Day 2 of 7

Date: _____ Day 3 of 7

Date: _____ Day 4 of 7

Date: _____ Day 5 of 7

Date: _____ Day 6 of 7

Date: _____ Day 7 of 7 ☺

24. Our Children

The adage "it takes a village to raise a child" echoes the truth. Children need attention, guidance, patience, instruction, emotional regulation, and nurturing. In return, they give their villages many gifts: their squeals of laughter, otherworldly thought processing, trust, or even their wariness offer new insights.

We know children are impressionable, but we cannot understand the full impact of our words on them. Why not leave them with positive affirmations?

Tell a child in your community how special they are. Try to think beyond outward appearance. Watch their actions and encourage them about them. If they are talkative, say they are gifted communicators. If they are always dancing, dance with them and celebrate their talent. Highlight intelligence or strength. Encourage them, as you would a friend, and help them recognize their greatness.

For this week, write about notable comments you received as a child—whether positive or negative. Describe the responses of the children you encouraged.

Date: _____ Day 1 of 7

Date: _____ Day 2 of 7

Date: _____ Day 3 of 7

Date: _____ Day 4 of 7

Date: _____ Day 5 of 7

Date: _____ Day 6 of 7

Date: _____ Day 7 of 7 ☺

25. Focus on Objects

Many societies are saturated with consumerism. We work hard to buy items we need but often get more that we simply want. After all that effort to obtain objects, what do we know about them?

For the next seven days, look for objects in your environment to explore. It could be plants outside or objects in the home. Try not to harm plants in this exercise. Safely engage with an item per day with all of your senses.

Be as a child with it. Stare at it for a minute from all angles. What do you see? Does it have a smell? Is there a texture? Imagine how it might taste. Notice something new about the item. Write your observations.

Share your discoveries with loved ones. Appreciate that you get to focus and learn about something—whether it be ordinary or extraordinary.

Date: _____ Day 1 of 7

Item:

Date: _____ Day 2 of 7

Item:

Date: _____ Day 3 of 7

Item:

Date: _____ Day 4 of 7

Item:

Date: _____ Day 5 of 7

Item:

Date: _____ Day 6 of 7

Item:

Date: _____ Day 7 of 7 ☺

Item:

26. Rest Daily

We start sleeping most of the day as infants. Over time, we whittle away at the hours we use for rest. No matter what age, sleep remains essential. Our functioning compacity is compromised when we neglect rest. It may impact us physically, emotionally, and socially to be tired.

The average adult should achieve a minimum of seven hours of sleep, ideally in the evenings. Are you meeting that mark? If not, what is preventing you from achieving it?

Consider your sleeping area. Do you have a comfortable resting place in a peaceful environment? Are you bringing distractions into your resting place? What is keeping you from offering your brain, which is always on for you, this time of rejuvenation?

For the next seven days, as far as it is within your power, get at least seven hours of continuous sleep. Try different tactics to achieve this. Peers and health providers may offer advice. (Sleep hygiene is a popular subject that is searchable online.)

Write about the benefits of sleep and what keeps you up at night. How does a lack of sleep change your day?

Date: _____ Day 1 of 7

Date: _____ Day 2 of 7

Date: _____ Day 3 of 7

Date: _____ Day 4 of 7

Date: _____ Day 5 of 7

Date: _____ Day 6 of 7

Date: _____ Day 7 of 7 ☺

27. Eat Vegetables

Food nurtures the mind. Choosing the right foods makes a difference in how you feel and think. This week, focus on eating more vegetables. Select a variety of root, leafy, sweet, or bitter vegetables to incorporate into your meals. There are so many gifts of the Earth to explore. What better way to understand how we enjoy nourishing our bodies than to try different options?

Look for recipes online. Try boiled, sauteed, spiralized, or steamed vegetables. Ask friends about their favorite vegetables. (I like to lump nuts, beans, and seeds with vegetables. Try quinoa. Try chia seeds in dairy or dairy substitutes. Experiment with different nuts as tolerated.)

Write your plans and discoveries. Which vegetable did you try? Did you enjoy any cooking techniques or dishes? What vegetables might you consider keeping in your diet? How is exploring these options changing what you are considering for your health?

Date: _____ Day 1 of 7

Date: _____ Day 2 of 7

Date: _____ Day 3 of 7

Date: _____ Day 4 of 7

Date: _____ Day 5 of 7

Date: _____ Day 6 of 7

Date: _____ Day 7 of 7 ☺

28. Dance Daily

Music surrounds us. From simple breaths to melodies vibrating against our eardrums, it often inspires us to motion.

Dance is often associated with celebration or art. Life is worth celebrating; to have life is to have something priceless.

Celebrate where possible today and for the next six days by moving your body to music. It may help to try a new form of dance and practice it daily.

Make sure you use a lot of space with your movements. Buy into the celebration.

Write about your favorite music. Why do you like it? What are your opinions on dance? Is there an artist or genre of music that makes you want to dance?

Date: _____ Day 1 of 7

Date: _____ Day 2 of 7

Date: _____ Day 3 of 7

Date: _____ Day 4 of 7

Date: _____ Day 5 of 7

Date: _____ Day 6 of 7

Date: _____ Day 7 of 7 ☺

29. Share Love

Consider the moon. It illuminates the night sky and morphs into different shapes over time. It glitters over and surprises us with its colors or disappearance. Yet, it's not by its own light that it shines.

No one is an island. We all have benefited from those who nurture and support us.

Who comes to mind when you think of love, encouragement, joy, peace, hope, strength, generosity, intelligence, and wisdom?

Contact a special person in your life daily and share something that you like or love about them. It could be a call or message. It could also be an acquaintance (if done politely). Tell those around you that you recognize how their presence builds up your life.

Write about the positive people in your life. Who did you contact? Was their response surprising? How often do you share your feelings with those in your life?

Date: _____ Day 1 of 7

Date: _____ Day 2 of 7

Date: _____ Day 3 of 7

Date: _____ Day 4 of 7

Date: _____ Day 5 of 7

Date: _____ Day 6 of 7

Date: _____ Day 7 of 7 ☺

30. Good News Only

Acorn seeds don't produce apples. Similarly, swarming our minds with negative imagery and chaos seeds can only produce more of the same. To live well, curate an environment of peace for yourself.

Distance yourself from what drains you. Turn off negativity. Avoid watching news reports. Stay off social media (if there is constant negativity there). Instead, focus on things that spark joy and reflect love.

If you want to fill that space, find media that makes you curious, laugh, and smile. Search for books, music, or encouraging videos. Think along the lines of animals, heartwarming stories, or comedies.

For the next seven days, protect your space and allow only those people, media, or tasks that promote emotions you desire to enter your realm. It can be challenging to revamp habits, but you deserve peace and joy.

Write about what it takes to prioritize the positive. What are some of your favorite items and activities? Who are some of your favorite people?

Date: _____ Day 1 of 7

Date: _____ Day 2 of 7

Date: _____ Day 3 of 7

Date: _____ Day 4 of 7

Date: _____ Day 5 of 7

Date: _____ Day 6 of 7

Date: _____ Day 7 of 7 ☺

31. Notice Your Body

As newborns, we weigh just a few pounds, barely occupying space. Then, there is rapid growth that eventually slows and plateaus. Our bodies have endured much over the years. Yet while being, they do everything for us. Bones shape us. Muscles move us. We may never fully understand how our bodies serve us, but that doesn't negate our ability to appreciate it.

This week, consider the functions that your body supports. Spend each day looking at a different part of your body. Set a timer for 1-2 minutes minimum and stare. Acknowledge that part is yours and working for you.

Notice the details. Are there marks or scars? Do they have memories attached? Thank your body. Are your features shared with someone you know? What is your favorite physical feature? Why? Write.

Date: _____ Day 1 of 7

Date: _____ Day 2 of 7

Date: _____ Day 3 of 7

Date: _____ Day 4 of 7

Date: _____ Day 5 of 7

Date: _____ Day 6 of 7

Date: _____ Day 7 of 7 ☺

32. Gift Giving

We think of gifts during special occasions—Christmas, birthdays, weddings, baby showers, and graduations. Yet, it is possible to find something to celebrate daily. There are people, events, milestones, and miracles every day. We ought to honor those.

Living generously is part of living well. A scarcity mindset detracts from relationships with self and others. For healthier relationships, foster a lifestyle of abundance.

For this week, be creative about giving gifts. If you go to an event, consider bringing an item the group would like. If you see a friend, surprise them with a small treat. Gifts do not need to have a price tag. Time is also a gift. Volunteer to help someone with a challenging task.

Living generously is about being present for others. They notice the thoughtfulness. Giving always pays off.

Write about your plans to give and times when you received meaningful help. As you give, consider the responses. How does it feel to be a giver?

Date: _____ Day 1 of 7

Date: _____ Day 2 of 7

Date: _____ Day 3 of 7

Date: _____ Day 4 of 7

Date: _____ Day 5 of 7

Date: _____ Day 6 of 7

Date: _____ Day 7 of 7 ☺

33. Wealth in Water

Water makes up more than half of our bodies, flowing through our cells and systems. The constant flow allows our bodies to survive. Water fills any container and floats out into the air. It surrounds us. It falls from the sky as ice, flakes, or droplets. The regular consumption and loss of water make it feel ordinary, but not much else is as incredible as water that holds and sustains life.

For the next seven days, pay attention to the amount of water you drink. Plan a safe activity with water and reflect on its essentiality. Walk near water, visit an aquarium or waterpark, or swim. (If you cannot swim, consider taking swimming lessons.) Try something unique.

What is your favorite use of water? What can you do to optimize water consumption? Write about what water allows you to do. Have you traveled by water? What bodies of water have you seen? What are some secrets held by water? Express your gratitude for the many roles of water in your life.

Date: _____

How much water will you drink each day?

Plan for water related activity:

Date: _____ Day 2 of 7

Did you drink your target amount of water?

Date: _____ Day 3 of 7

Did you drink your target amount of water?

Date: _____ Day 4 of 7

Did you drink your target amount of water?

Date: _____ Day 5 of 7

Did you drink your target amount of water?

Date: _____ Day 6 of 7

Did you drink your target amount of water?

Date: _____ Day 7 of 7 ☺

Did you drink your target amount of water?

34. Sleep Well

Routines, aside from adding order to life, may be comforting. They offer consistency and something to look forward to, particularly in chaotic situations. Routines, when disrupted, also signal that a reset is needed. One timeless routine is sleeping. It should happen every day. The evenings herald the time for rest. Are we regularly answering the call of our circadian rhythms?

For the next seven days, sleep and wake at the same time. Plan for your time of sleep. Remove distractions from your resting place. Set and adhere to boundaries. Determine how you will wake up and what you will do before sleeping.

What are some of your routines? Were there times when they were disrupted? Why? How did you return to your baseline? What benefits do they add to your life? Are there routines you want to incorporate into your schedule for your well-being? What steps would help you to achieve your hopes? What causes you to lose sleep? Consistent and adequate rest is essential to wellness. Prioritizing rest is part of success.

Date: _____ Day 1 of 7

| Sleep time: |
| Wake time: |
| What will you do to prepare for sleep? |

Date: _____ Day 2 of 7

Date: _____ Day 3 of 7

Date: _____ Day 4 of 7

Date: _____ Day 5 of 7

Date: _____ Day 6 of 7

Date: _____ Day 7 of 7 ☺

35. Celebrate Life

For months we are incubated in a womb; all that we are is dependent on another. Then suddenly we are squeezed out into the world. How incredible is it to be born—to now have a name. To start breathing and experiencing a new realm individually.

This week, consider the gift of existence. (Perhaps you choose this exercise around your birthday week?) Get or make a gift to acknowledge that you have another day. Wear and eat something special. Make plans that will bring you joy. Take time off to celebrate and rest.

Think about some benefits of living and give thanks for them. Who gives you the most support? Consider how you have changed. Write about your gratitude and how far you have come. Write about your favorite memories. Are there people who changed the trajectory of your life? Were you present for someone's birth? How was that experience? Write about your birthday or other celebrations.

Date: _____ Day 1 of 7

Date: _____ Day 2 of 7

Date: _____ Day 3 of 7

Date: _____ Day 4 of 7

Date: _____ Day 5 of 7

Date: _____ Day 6 of 7

Date: _____ Day 7 of 7 ☺

36. Be With Friends

Have you ever found yourself in a restaurant, watching people more focused on their phones than their companions? Or have you attended a party and noticed people using technology to avoid socializing? These days, we have so many options for distractions, but not all of them are good. Though technology has advanced to connect people, it is easier now to choose worthless distractions over valuable connections.

Building relationships requires quality time studying someone to understand if you might fit into their lives. It necessitates identifying common interests and areas where you might build together.

We must stay in the present moment to reap the benefits of relationships and put aside what will always be accessible.

For the next week, while you are with people, avoid social media. Be intentional with family, friends, co-workers, or even someone new (who is safe and interesting). Learn about their hobbies, dreams, and current fascinations. Learn about who has influenced them and where they hope to be in their next chapter. Share your story.

Reflect on the finite moments you spend with people. What are differences between in-person and virtual communications? How have your relationships shaped your decisions and life? Consider your close circle. Are you around people who inspire you?

Date: _____ Day 1 of 7

Date: _____ Day 2 of 7

Date: _____ Day 3 of 7

Date: _____ Day 4 of 7

Date: _____ Day 5 of 7

Date: _____ Day 6 of 7

Date: _____ Day 7 of 7 ☺

37. Values

We exist because many factors were in perfect alignment. Yet, life is imperfect. There are unpredictable seasons and individuals that influence our path. While journeying through life, what is our guiding post?

We need values to make the right decisions for ourselves. Clear values serve as a foundation to support us, particularly in times of disorder.

Our values define our purpose. They influence relationships and the integrity of an individual.

For this week, identify 1-3 values and consider ways that your life reflects those values. Limited examples are below. (Consider exploring values online.) Each day create a new list of three values until you get up to 15 total. On day six, use your five previous lists to select values that resonate with you the most. Further narrow your list to three values by day seven.

Consider what occupies your thoughts, work that is meaningful to you, your fears, where you seek to improve, what motivates you through challenges, how you spend your time, and how you were raised when deciding on values.

Examples of Values			
Excellence	Joy	Peace	Confidence
Generosity	Service	Unity	Justice
Loyalty	Honesty	Faith/Spirituality	Leadership
Reliability	Honor	Beauty	Wealth
Learning	Respect	Growth	Empathy
Wisdom	Family	Adventure/Fun	Support
Originality	Recognition	Courage	Tradition
Intelligence	Love	Achievement	Selflessness
Adaptability	Tradition	Health	Reflection
Independence	Prosperity	Philanthropy	Integrity
Safety	Creativity	Discipline	Strength

Date: _____ Day 1 of 7

Choose 3 values and reflect on how they show up in your life

1.
2.
3.

Date: _____ Day 2 of 7

Choose 3 new values and reflect on how they show up in your life

1.
2.
3.

Date: _____ Day 3 of 7

Choose 3 new values and reflect on how they show up in your life

1.
2.
3.

Date: _____ Day 4 of 7

Choose 3 new values and reflect on how they show up in your life

1.
2.
3.

Date: _____ Day 5 of 7

Choose 3 new values and reflect on how they show up in your life

1. _____
2. _____
3. _____

Date: _____ Day 6 of 7

Use the previous lists to select the most meaningful values

1. _____
2. _____
3. _____
4. _____
5. _____
6. _____
7. _____
8. _____

Date: _____ Day 7 of 7 ☺

What are your 3 values?

1.
2.
3.

38. In the Clouds

When the sun creeps out of hiding, it illuminates the world and lets us see the clouds. Not everyone gets to experience the light of the sun daily. (For one example, ask our Alaskan friends.) What a gift is the consistency of the sun.

Clouds are less predictable. The sky might be clear or peppered with white/gray shapes waiting for our imagination to sort out. Take time during the day to watch the sky. (Avoid looking directly into the sun.)

If clouds are there, look for shapes in them. Draw the shapes. Tell stories that give the shapes meaning. Maybe the clouds remind you of someone you can share your thoughts with? Can you imagine touching them? How might they feel? What about the difference you see when flying amongst them on a plane?

(Try deciphering trees, plants, or rocks if there is no luck in the cloud department.)

Date: _____ Day 1 of 7

Date: _____ Day 2 of 7

Date: _____ Day 3 of 7

Date: _____ Day 4 of 7

Date: _____ Day 5 of 7

Date: _____ Day 6 of 7

Date: _____ Day 7 of 7 ☺

39. Great Gifts

Have you ever given a gift so thoughtful that you saw the receiver's demeanor shift at the sight of it? Or maybe you received a special present? Do you remember how it felt to have it? Was it a surprise?

Gifts come in various forms. They don't have to cost much to be meaningful. Time shared is also a gift.

For the next 7 days, think about memorable gifts you received, whether they were for a special occasion or not. Write about why the gift is special to you. Who gave you the gift? What was the first moment with it like? Do the feelings return at the thought? Did you take pictures with your gift? Is that person still accessible? If you feel inclined, contact the gifter and share your thanks again.

Date: _____ Day 1 of 7

Date: _____ Day 2 of 7

Date: _____ Day 3 of 7

Date: _____ Day 4 of 7

Date: _____ Day 5 of 7

Date: _____ Day 6 of 7

Date: _____ Day 7 of 7 ☺

40. Exercise

At birth, we received what cannot be bought nor replaced. We get one body and are tasked to care for it as best as we know how. Fortunately, we can increase our know-how. It can be fun to strive for wellness. Many options will achieve the same goal.

For the next seven days, try a new form of exercise. It could be a unique one daily or a few days during the week that you try an exercise plan. There are many ways to get moving—swim, jump rope, Pilates, Zumba, and other dances. Hydrate and exercise for at least 30 minutes per day. Recruit friends for advice (if needed).

Write about your time exercising. Is the exercise fun? Are there ways to make it more engaging? Are you creating challenges for yourself to meet? Did you take breaks? Are you drinking enough water? Celebrate small wins and dream about health gains to make exercising more rewarding.

Date: _____ Day 1 of 7

Exercise plan:

Date: _____ Day 2 of 7

Date: _____ Day 3 of 7

Date: _____ Day 4 of 7

Date: _____ Day 5 of 7

Date: _____ Day 6 of 7

Date: _____ Day 7 of 7 ☺

41. Self-Forgiveness

Each day offers new benefits and challenges. How we choose to respond to them shapes our experiences. Did we plan for success or stumble into failure? Sometimes, due to our choices, we need to forgive ourselves. Immature expressions of anger, hurtful words, broken promises, or neglecting to put our best foot forward to achieve a goal can leave us with remorse.

For this exercise, consider something personal that may require forgiveness. It could be big or small. Write about one instance daily and an alternate course of action you could take to avoid similar outcomes in the future.

A good place to start may be considering memories that make you feel regret—those memories that curdle your stomach when you think about them. Perhaps you are now in a situation that stems from a past choice or behavior.

Identify these moments. Write them. Say, "I forgive myself," even if it is not true yet. You don't have to keep the words. Particularly if they induce negative emotions. You can destroy them or draw a beautiful picture over them as a symbol of letting what holds you back go. Forgiveness gives freedom. You deserve to feel free.

Date: _____ Day 1 of 7

Date: _____ Day 2 of 7

Date: _____ Day 3 of 7

Date: _____ Day 4 of 7

Date: _____ Day 5 of 7

Date: _____ Day 6 of 7

Date: _____ Day 7 of 7 ☺

42. Smiles

A smile is an obvious sign of warmth and positivity. Smiles are gifts. They can shift the mood in the room. Smiling is contagious. In times of difficulty, we often realize how precious they are. But the Earth holds many gifts for us. Using our imaginations, we can see them in unexpected places.

For the next 7 days, look for smiles (or faces) in ordinary objects. Point them out to others. Write about where you found them. Did the discovery change your perspective? Did you smile back? Write.

Date: _____ Day 1 of 7

Date: _____ Day 2 of 7

Date: _____ Day 3 of 7

Date: _____ Day 4 of 7

Date: _____ Day 5 of 7

Date: _____ Day 6 of 7

Date: _____ Day 7 of 7 ☺

43. Sense of Thanks

Every day we engage with the world using our senses of smell, sight, hearing, taste, touch, etc. Senses teach us. Our minds process that complex information. Our organs work without conscious input on our part. Not everyone has every ability, and those who lose a sense recognize this keenly.

Take time daily to thank your senses. Do it throughout the day or choose a time to sit and reflect on how your senses serve you. Take a moment to savor a delicious taste. If you are admiring something beautiful, thank your eyes for their ability to see. If you are enjoying a soft texture, be thankful for your skin.

Write about the advantages gained through senses. Can you think of an animal that senses the world differently? Is there an ability you wish you had? Imagine what you would do with that ability.

Date: _____ Day 1 of 7

Date: _____ Day 2 of 7

Date: _____ Day 3 of 7

Date: _____ Day 4 of 7

Date: _____ Day 5 of 7

Date: _____ Day 6 of 7

Date: _____ Day 7 of 7 ☺

44. Eat for Enrichment

Eating a diet of fruits, vegetables, low-sodium food, minimal sugar, and healthy fats could change a life. But where do you begin? Try seven days of experimenting with NEW fruits, vegetables, meat alternatives, and healthier oils. Talk to a dietitian or explore a Mediterranean diet for ideas.

Throughout and particularly at the end of seven days, reflect on whether this healthier option can be added to your habits, how you feel, what you learned, and how your body is working.

How is your diet? What do you eat a lot of? Where do you get most of your food? How often do you eat a hot meal? What would be your ideal diet? What keeps you from eating to support your health?

Date: _____ Day 1 of 7

Date: _____ Day 2 of 7

Date: _____ Day 3 of 7

Date: _____ Day 4 of 7

Date: _____ Day 5 of 7

Date: _____ Day 6 of 7

Date: _____ Day 7 of 7 ☺

45. Greet Yourself

A nod, a smile, a hug, a kind word—there are countless ways to greet people. It is a social policy when meeting someone to acknowledge their presence. But we meet ourselves daily and treat that as commonplace.

Let's be more polite to ourselves. You are your most faithful companion. The only one guaranteed to be physically present in life. How do you acknowledge yourself? Are your thoughts kind, encouraging, patient, loving, or peaceful?

If you want to guide yourself to more favorable thoughts, you could start with one tangible and familiar act. Greet yourself. Look in a mirror. Smile and try out different greetings when you start your day. Then you will always know that someone is happy to see you.

Consider greetings that you have seen or received. Which ones stand out? Was it a hug or an expression that made it meaningful? Write about your favorite greetings.

Date: _____ Day 1 of 7

Date: _____ Day 2 of 7

Date: _____ Day 3 of 7

Date: _____ Day 4 of 7

Date: _____ Day 5 of 7

Date: _____ Day 6 of 7

Date: _____ Day 7 of 7 ☺

46. Reframe the Negative

The Earth is estimated to be over four billion years old. For all the time humans have roamed it, they had challenges. It is a universal part of life to reckon with a unique set of circumstances that shape us. There is nothing new under the sun, but the sun keeps shining.

In tough situations, it may be difficult to see the silver lining; particularly if it is the first challenge. The first encounter with death, illness, or failure is especially devastating. Yet, what can this new experience nurture? Does a death evoke an appreciation for the precious time shared? Does illness enhance recollections of wellness or empathy for others? Does failure revamp plans and hope for the future?

Challenges are signals for growth. With time distancing us from adversity, it is often easier to see the positive changes wrought by the devastation. But why wait to reap the benefits?

Though challenging, it is possible to reframe a negative to help you move forward. It is possible to consider career setbacks as opportunities to pivot towards purpose. It is possible to see the end of a relationship as creating space for someone who wants to add value to your life.

For the next week, consider a negative situation that changed your perspective or position in life. Negative experiences could be relatively slight too, such as an interaction with a stranger or an academic mishap. Reflect on one instance per day and write about the new insights. Gratitude may arise from reframing the past, but it doesn't have to.

Out of something devastating, find the light.

Date: _____ Day 1 of 7

Date: _____ Day 2 of 7

Date: _____ Day 3 of 7

Date: _____ Day 4 of 7

Date: _____ Day 5 of 7

Date: _____ Day 6 of 7

Date: _____ Day 7 of 7 ☺

47. Play Daily

There are seasons in life that require changes. Whether it is to accommodate people, careers, or health.

Some folks remember childhood or youth as a phenomenal season. What made that season so special? Was it the time playing with friends and loved ones?

There is no reason to stop playing as adults. If we are fortunate, we still have people around us who love us and want to participate in fun activities.

Suggestions are game nights, make-shift obstacle courses, tag, or hide-and-seek. Set positive goals for each game, such as laughing or cheering more.

Even if only for 15 minutes per day, make time to play. If living independently, seek games like hula hoop, hopscotch, swinging, or chess with opponents online.

Write about the games chosen. Was it active? Did you win? How much did you laugh?

Date: _____ Day 1 of 7

Date: _____ Day 2 of 7

Date: _____ Day 3 of 7

Date: _____ Day 4 of 7

Date: _____ Day 5 of 7

Date: _____ Day 6 of 7

Date: _____ Day 7 of 7 ☺

48. Purposeful Reading

Flamingos, with their tall scrawny legs and enviable one-legged balance, develop feathery robes in various shades of pink. Interestingly, it is what they choose to eat that gives them their signature color.

Similar to our feathery colleagues, we are what we consume. There are countless fresh, encouraging, fascinating, inspiring, comical, and joyful ideas. In the time we have, we will barely scratch the surface, particularly if we are not searching for the good and true.

During the next week, choose a book that aligns with your personal development goals or is enjoyable. Commit to reading for at least 30 minutes per day.

Reflect on why you chose your source. Was it a recommendation? Are you familiar with the author? Does it have an engaging title? Is it meeting your expectations? How do you feel about the cover of the book? Are there new ideas for you to explore? Write.

Date: _____ Day 1 of 7

Title of your book:

Date: _____ Day 2 of 7

Date: _____ Day 3 of 7

Date: _____ Day 4 of 7

Date: _____ Day 5 of 7

Date: _____ Day 6 of 7

Date: _____ Day 7 of 7 ☺

49. Ask It

When we look in the mirror, what do we see? Our reflection is shaped by our biases. Our perception of ourselves differs from how others see us because they view us based on their unique life experiences. The only way to know the difference is to ask.

For friendly acquaintances and people you value, it may help to understand how they perceive you. Ask them: What do you appreciate about me? How can I improve as a sibling, co-worker, partner, etc.? What do you think of when you think of me?

You may be surprised by what people will say in a private conversation. Asking good questions gives you an idea of what skills you should strengthen or work towards adjusting for stronger relationships.

Find a person to ask these questions daily. Reflect on their responses. Are they consistent? What unique responses did you get? Do you resonate with what was shared? What areas do you hope to work on? Write about what you learn.

Date: _____ Day 1 of 7

Date: _____ Day 2 of 7

Date: _____ Day 3 of 7

Date: _____ Day 4 of 7

Date: _____ Day 5 of 7

Date: _____ Day 6 of 7

Date: _____ Day 7 of 7 ☺

50. Positive Routine

The sun rises and sets every day (for most of us). Yet the beauty evoked by the sun's motion can still captivate. There is something comforting about routines. They serve as a light at the end of a tunnel. In the night, we know the day will come. During the day, there is hope of greeting the moon.

The Earth and sun gave us routines as examples of what is useful to implement for ourselves.

Think of an encouraging, enriching, or health-improving routine to follow for the next seven days. Have a plan. Choose a time that you can do your routine consistently. Consider pairing the new activity with something you regularly do as a reminder. (Think: After I brush my teeth, I will meditate for five minutes.)

Some examples are self-care regimes, daily accountability meetings, stock market monitoring, or calling different family members. It helps to have a goal in mind—whether it's advancing your career, deepening your relationships, or growing spiritually. Claim the goal as yours daily, then make a small step towards it.

Reflect on why your routine has meaning. Think about your emotions each day. If you come to your routine time with negative feelings, set them aside to focus on what is positive and intended for your benefit. Write.

Date: _____ Day 1 of 7

Date: _____ Day 2 of 7

Date: _____ Day 3 of 7

Date: _____ Day 4 of 7

Date: _____ Day 5 of 7

Date: _____ Day 6 of 7

Date: _____ Day 7 of 7 ☺

51. Sleep Grateful

Earth is spinning, spinning, spinning 24 hours a day. For some, 24 hours is too much, and for others, not enough. Working or caring for other responsibilities consumes our hours before we sleep.

What is your attitude when you sleep? Is it one that you would like to stay with you throughout your next day? Can you instead choose to reflect on what you are thankful for as you are lulled into rest?

Reflect on five things you are grateful for before sleeping. Why do you value them? If it is too distracting to write as you go to sleep, write about your appreciation and how you felt as you wake.

Date: _____ Day 1 of 7

1.
2.
3.
4.
5.

Date: _____ Day 2 of 7

1.
2.
3.
4.
5.

Date: _____ Day 3 of 7

1.
2.
3.
4.
5.

Date: _____ Day 4 of 7

1.
2.
3.
4.
5.

Date: _____ Day 5 of 7

1.
2.
3.
4.
5.

Date: _____ Day 6 of 7

1.
2.
3.
4.
5.

Date: _____ Day 7 of 7 ☺

1.
2.
3.
4.
5.

52. Celebrate Success

In the background of the horizon, mountains sit. Holding a myriad of secrets and adventures for those who seek them. Though daunting, even the tallest mountains on Earth were climbed. They are conquerable, and we are conquerors.

We all face obstacles—some that appear looming. We know the resources and support it takes to move past them. It may feel like we face them alone, but when we emerge from battles, there is usually someone on the other side.

Take this week to be on the leeward side of the mountain and celebrate the successes of others. Do for others as you hope someone will do for you.

Success looks different to each person. If they share it with you or the world, match or exceed their enthusiasm. If you find success on social media, share encouragement. If you see someone celebrating, add your well wishes. Reflect on how they have grown, conquered, achieved, shared, loved, or believed.

Write about a personal success daily. Write about how it felt to encourage others. What inspired you about their accomplishments? Searching for avenues to encourage success in others will help you to identify personal triumphs.

Date: _____ Day 1 of 7

Date: _____ Day 2 of 7

Date: _____ Day 3 of 7

Date: _____ Day 4 of 7

Date: _____ Day 5 of 7

Date: _____ Day 6 of 7

Date: _____ Day 7 of 7 ☺

PART III

Conclusion

Though the exercises may be at an end, your journey to purpose is only beginning. Continue refining your values and prioritizing what matters—relationships, character, generosity, peace, health, emotional resilience, etc. Enrich your life by finding reasons to celebrate, appreciate, and love those around you. Keep your childlike wonder. Protect your peace. Nurture habits that draw you closer to contentment. Give grace to yourself as well as to others.

While hardships are inevitable, your response to them is controllable. Release mindsets that hinder your growth. Maintain your worth and power to move past challenges and come out healthier. Your behavior should not be controlled by circumstances or those around you. Feel every emotion but don't let feelings hold or move you. Use your values to guide your actions. No matter the situation, never accept the identity of a failure. You may fail at tasks, but if you continue, you are on the path to success.

Remember the divinity in each moment. Make time to cherish and grow from your experiences. Plan to explore the world. Life has countless gifts waiting for you. Shift your perspective to find the fun, hope, beauty, excellence, strength, and joy in everything. When you develop habits that align with your health goals and purpose, you will have more than an intentional year—you will have a phenomenal life.

Alternatives

a. Color Daily

Our universe is a canvas of vibrant colors. Spectacular hues made known to us in the light. It is a gift to see them.

Let us celebrate colors for the next seven days by using them to complete a picture. Each day draw and color a picture. Try different tools such as paint, markers, pens, or crayons.

Alternatively, you can use the first day of the week to choose your favorite images online or purchase them in a store. (The remaining days would be for coloring.) Make it fun. Consider picking a theme.

Write your reflections on your day and the image. Notice the kind of paper you are coloring. Is it glossy? Thin? How does your tool feel running across it? Does it glide smoothly? What else do you notice?

b. Laugh Daily

Laughter is medicine. Even in tragic situations a laugh can shift the whole atmosphere. It is particularly in unfortunate circumstances that we might realize how sacred laughter is. Oftentimes the memories that stay fresh are those that evoke or involve laughter. It is one of life's most salient gifts.

Consider who or what makes you laugh the most. How do you feel about that subject? Does it add to your life? Write.

For the next seven days, make an effort to laugh two times a day. Start right now. No reason is necessary. If it helps to have one, seek out people who are funny or known comical sources.

c. Turtle Detection

Imagine carrying your home everywhere you go. Turtles amble around with their attached shells, and do not let the myth that they are slow fool you. (I once saw a turtle running through a parking lot.) They live in versatile habitats but—especially if you live in wet or swampy areas with various bodies of water—you may be lucky enough to spot them.

If you walk by a body of water, look for the flat round reptiles. You may see their little heads poke out of the water. They sometimes commune on a log or rock. Other times turtles are catching sun on the edge of water. Make it a game to find them and watch them live their best lives.

Alternatively, you can go to a zoo or a pet store and observe the animals there. Another option is to watch animal videos or movies. Reflect on how the animals you see live their lives. What is different and intriguing?

d. Dream Daily

When was the last time your mind took you on exotic adventures? Most of us sleep every day, but when was the last time we had a dream wherein we conquered, found treasure, discovered, and celebrated?

Dreams can be realized. We can build a life for ourselves that is worth discussing. The first step in doing so is to create the idea. The details may be too extensive to encapsulate in a picture.

What would you do if possibilities were limitless? Where would you go? How would you live? What kind of person would you be? What would you wear? Envisioning possibilities builds hope. Hope enriches the mind.

Write and speak your dreams daily to encourage yourself and explore excellent possibilities. Try to dream aloud for at least 10 minutes. Fill in all the details. Dream big and include all your favorites in the vision. Bring it to life.

Acknowledgements

I am grateful for my parents whose boundless ingenuity and resilience shaped me. To my friends, some of whom reviewed chapters, thank you for the love and consistency you have shown me. To my nieces, nephews, and every child I have guided, you are the lights of my life. I pray that you discover a love that is unfathomable.

To my siblings, who keep me laughing and who are models of level-headedness, I look forward to the legacy we will build. To COOL Church and the B2B group, God was looking out for me with these connections.

To the people of the Memoir Writing Workshop, I am so grateful to sit and listen to a room full of wisdom and to share some of my story with you. To my readers, thank you for contributing to a dream come true.

Most significantly, I give glory to God who has granted me a greater life than I could ever imagine and whose provision of ideas, education, and peace has seen me through the toughest of trials.

About the Author

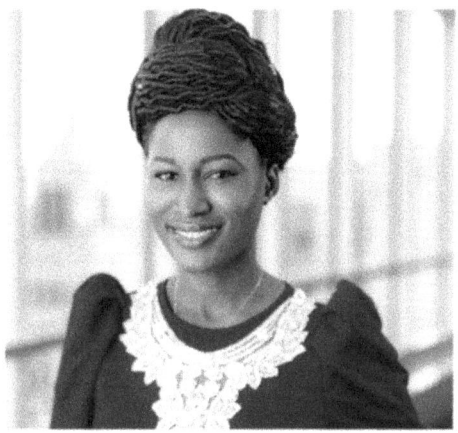

Dr. Josiane Joseph is a dreamer, speaker, author, physician, scientist, entrepreneur, blogger, and educator dedicated to building healthier communities. As the founder of Double Doc J LLC, she collaborates with groups and individuals to develop a mindset that supports them in planning for and expecting success.

Along the way, she earned a PhD in Clinical and Translational Science (exploring skeletal muscle regeneration), an MD, a BS in Biology, and an AA in Business Administration. Each step of her academic path was fueled by a desire to make a lasting impact.

Beyond her professional endeavors, Dr. Joseph enjoys traveling, attending theater performances, hiking, and nurturing meaningful relationships. She credits much of her personal and professional success to relationships rooted in her core values of joy, love, and growth.

Connect with Dr. Joseph:
DoubleDocJ.com
◎ DoubleDocJ

www.ingramcontent.com/pod-product-compliance
Lightning Source LLC
Chambersburg PA
CBHW060448030426
42337CB00015B/1521